AF499246

Table of Contents

Introduction

Cancer is a group of diseases involving abnormal cell growth with the potential to invade or spread to other parts of the body. These contrast with benign tumors, which do not spread. Possible signs and symptoms include a lump, abnormal bleeding, prolonged cough, unexplained weight loss, and a change in bowel movements. While these symptoms may indicate cancer, they can also have other causes. Over 100 types of cancers affect humans.

Tobacco use is the cause of about 22% of cancer deaths. Another 10% are due to obesity, poor diet, lack of physical activity or excessive drinking of alcohol. Other factors include certain infections, exposure to ionizing radiation, and environmental pollutants. In the developing world, 15% of cancers are due to infections such as Helicobacter pylori, hepatitis B, hepatitis C, human papillomavirus infection, Epstein–Barr virus and human immunodeficiency virus (HIV). These factors act, at least partly, by changing the genes of a cell. Typically, many genetic changes are required before cancer develops. Approximately 5–10% of cancers are due to inherited genetic defects. Cancer can be detected by certain signs and symptoms or screening tests. It is then typically further investigated by medical imaging and confirmed by biopsy.

The risk of developing certain cancers can be reduced by not smoking, maintaining a healthy weight, limiting alcohol intake, eating plenty of vegetables, fruits, and whole grains, vaccination against certain infectious diseases, limiting consumption of processed meat and red meat, and limiting exposure to direct sunlight. Early detection through screening is useful for cervical and colorectal cancer. The benefits of screening in breast cancer are controversial. Cancer is often treated with some combination of radiation therapy, surgery, chemotherapy and targeted therapy. Pain and symptom management are an important part of care. Palliative care is particularly important in people with advanced disease. The chance of survival depends on the type of cancer and extent of disease at the start of treatment. In children under 15 at diagnosis, the five-year survival rate in the developed world is on average 80%. For cancer in the United States, the average five-year survival rate is 66%.

In 2015, about 90.5 million people had cancer. As of 2019, about 18 million new cases occur annually. Annually, it caused about 8.8 million deaths (15.7% of deaths). The most common types of cancer in males are lung cancer, prostate cancer, colorectal cancer, and stomach cancer. In females, the most common types are breast cancer, colorectal cancer, lung cancer, and cervical cancer. If skin cancer other than melanoma were included in total new cancer cases each year, it would account for around 40% of cases. In children, acute lymphoblastic leukemia and brain tumors are most common, except in Africa, where non-Hodgkin lymphoma occurs more often. In 2012, about 165,000 children under 15 years of age were diagnosed with cancer. The risk of cancer increases significantly with age, and many cancers occur more commonly in developed countries. Rates are increasing as more people live to an old age and as lifestyle changes occur in the developing world. The financial costs of cancer were estimated at 1.16 trillion USD per year as of 2010.

Cancers comprise a large family of diseases that involve abnormal cell growth with the potential to invade or spread to other parts of the body. They form a subset of neoplasms. A neoplasm or tumor is a group of cells that have undergone unregulated growth and will often form a mass or lump, but may be distributed diffusely.

All tumor cells show the six hallmarks of cancer. These characteristics are required to produce a malignant tumor. They include:

- Cell growth and division absent the proper signals
- Continuous growth and division even given contrary signals
- Avoidance of programmed cell death
- Limitless number of cell divisions
- Promoting blood vessel construction
- Invasion of tissue and formation of metastases

- The progression from normal cells to cells that can form a detectable mass to outright cancer involves multiple steps known as malignant progression.

Signs and symptoms

When cancer begins, it produces no symptoms. Signs and symptoms appear as the mass grows or ulcerates. The findings that result depend on the cancer's type and location. Few symptoms are specific. Many frequently occur in individuals who have other conditions. Cancer can be difficult to diagnose and can be considered a "great imitator."

People may become anxious or depressed post-diagnosis. The risk of suicide in people with cancer is approximately double.

Local symptoms

Local symptoms may occur due to the mass of the tumor or its ulceration. For example, mass effects from lung cancer can block the bronchus resulting in cough or pneumonia; esophageal cancer can cause narrowing of the esophagus, making it difficult or painful to swallow; and colorectal cancer may lead to narrowing or blockages in the bowel, affecting bowel habits. Masses in breasts or testicles may produce observable lumps. Ulceration can cause bleeding that can lead to symptoms such as coughing up blood (lung cancer), anemia or rectal bleeding (colon cancer), blood in the urine (bladder cancer), or abnormal vaginal bleeding (endometrial or cervical cancer). Although localized pain may occur in advanced cancer, the initial tumor is usually painless. Some cancers can cause a buildup of fluid within the chest or abdomen.

Systemic symptoms

Systemic symptoms may occur due to the body's response to the cancer. This may include fatigue, unintentional weight loss, or skin changes. Some cancers can cause a systemic inflammatory state that leads to ongoing muscle loss and weakness, known as cachexia.

Some types of cancer such as Hodgkin disease, leukemias and cancers of the liver or kidney can cause a persistent fever.

Some systemic symptoms of cancer are caused by hormones or other molecules produced by the tumor, known as paraneoplastic syndromes. Common paraneoplastic syndromes include hypercalcemia which can cause altered mental state, constipation and dehydration, or hyponatremia that can also cause altered mental status, vomiting, headache or seizures.

Metastasis

Metastasis is the spread of cancer to other locations in the body. The dispersed tumors are called metastatic tumors, while the original is called the primary tumor. Almost all cancers can metastasize. Most cancer deaths are due to cancer that has metastasized.

Metastasis is common in the late stages of cancer and it can occur via the blood or the lymphatic system or both. The typical steps in metastasis are local invasion, intravasation into the blood or lymph, circulation through the body, extravasation into the new tissue, proliferation and angiogenesis. Different types of cancers tend to metastasize to particular organs, but overall the most common places for metastases to occur are the lungs, liver, brain and the bones.

Causes

The majority of cancers, some 90–95% of cases, are due to genetic mutations from environmental and lifestyle factors. The remaining 5–10% are due to inherited genetics. Environmental refers to any cause that is not inherited, such as lifestyle, economic, and behavioral factors and not merely pollution. Common environmental factors that contribute to cancer death include tobacco use (25–30%), diet and obesity (30–35%), infections (15–20%), radiation (both ionizing and non-ionizing, up to 10%), lack of physical activity, and pollution. Psychological stress does not appear to be a risk factor for the onset of cancer, though it may worsen outcomes in those who already have cancer.

It is not generally possible to prove what caused a particular cancer because the various causes do not have specific fingerprints. For example, if a person who uses tobacco heavily develops lung cancer, then it was probably caused by the tobacco use, but since everyone has a small chance of developing lung cancer as a result of air pollution or radiation, the cancer may have developed for one of those reasons. Excepting the rare transmissions that occur with pregnancies and occasional organ donors, cancer is generally not a transmissible disease.

Chemicals

The incidence of lung cancer is highly correlated with smoking.

Exposure to particular substances have been linked to specific types of cancer. These substances are called carcinogens.

Tobacco smoke, for example, causes 90% of lung cancer. It also causes cancer in the larynx, head, neck, stomach, bladder, kidney, esophagus and pancreas. Tobacco smoke contains over fifty known carcinogens, including nitrosamines and polycyclic aromatic hydrocarbons.

Tobacco is responsible for about one in five cancer deaths worldwide and about one in three in the developed world.

Lung cancer death rates in the United States have mirrored smoking patterns, with increases in smoking followed by dramatic increases in lung cancer death rates and, more recently, decreases in smoking rates since the 1950s followed by decreases in lung cancer death rates in men since 1990.

In Western Europe, 10% of cancers in males and 3% of cancers in females are attributed to alcohol exposure, especially liver and digestive tract cancers. Cancer from work-related substance exposures may cause between 2 and 20% of cases, causing at least 200,000 deaths. Cancers such as lung cancer and mesothelioma can come from inhaling tobacco smoke or asbestos fibers, or leukemia from exposure to benzene.

Diet and exercise

Diet, physical inactivity and obesity are related to up to 30–35% of cancer deaths. In the United States, excess body weight is associated with the development of many types of cancer and is a factor in 14–20% of cancer deaths. A UK study including data on over 5 million people showed higher body mass index to be related to at least 10 types of cancer and responsible for around 12,000 cases each year in that country. Physical inactivity is believed to contribute to cancer risk, not only through its effect on body weight but also through negative effects on the immune system and endocrine system. More than half of the effect from diet is due to overnutrition (eating too much), rather than from eating too few vegetables or other healthful foods.

Some specific foods are linked to specific cancers. A high-salt diet is linked to gastric cancer. Aflatoxin B1, a frequent food contaminant, causes liver cancer. Betel nut chewing can cause oral cancer. National differences in dietary practices may partly explain differences in cancer incidence. For example, gastric cancer is more common in Japan due to its high-salt diet while colon cancer is more common in the United States. Immigrant cancer profiles mirror those of their new country, often within one generation.

Infection

Worldwide approximately 18% of cancer deaths are related to infectious diseases. This proportion ranges from a high of 25% in Africa to less than 10% in the developed world. Viruses are the usual infectious agents that cause cancer but cancer bacteria and parasites may also play a role.

Oncoviruses (viruses that can cause cancer) include human papillomavirus (cervical cancer), Epstein–Barr virus (B-cell lymphoproliferative disease and nasopharyngeal carcinoma), Kaposi's sarcoma herpesvirus (Kaposi's sarcoma and primary effusion lymphomas), hepatitis B and hepatitis C viruses (hepatocellular carcinoma) and human T-cell leukemia virus-1 (T-cell leukemias). Bacterial infection may also increase the risk of cancer, as seen in Helicobacter pylori-induced gastric carcinoma. Parasitic infections associated with cancer include Schistosoma haematobium (squamous cell carcinoma of the bladder) and the liver flukes, Opisthorchis viverrini and Clonorchis sinensis (cholangiocarcinoma).

Radiation

Radiation exposure such as ultraviolet radiation and radioactive material is a risk factor for cancer. Many non-melanoma skin cancers are due to ultraviolet radiation, mostly from sunlight. Sources of ionizing radiation include medical imaging and radon gas.

Ionizing radiation is not a particularly strong mutagen. Residential exposure to radon gas, for example, has similar cancer risks as passive smoking. Radiation is a more potent source of cancer when combined with other cancer-causing agents, such as radon plus tobacco smoke. Radiation can cause cancer in most parts of the body, in all animals and at any age. Children are twice as likely to develop radiation-induced leukemia as adults; radiation exposure before birth has ten times the effect.

Medical use of ionizing radiation is a small but growing source of radiation-induced cancers. Ionizing radiation may be used to treat other cancers, but this may, in some cases, induce a second form of cancer. It is also used in some kinds of medical imaging.

Prolonged exposure to ultraviolet radiation from the sun can lead to melanoma and other skin malignancies. Clear evidence establishes ultraviolet radiation, especially the non-ionizing medium wave UVB, as the cause of most non-melanoma skin cancers, which are the most common forms of cancer in the world.

Non-ionizing radio frequency radiation from mobile phones, electric power transmission and other similar sources has been described as a possible carcinogen by the World Health Organization's International Agency for Research on Cancer. Evidence, however, has not supported a concern. This includes that studies have not found a consistent link between mobile phone radiation and cancer risk.

Heredity

The vast majority of cancers are non-hereditary (sporadic). Hereditary cancers are primarily caused by an inherited genetic defect. Less than 0.3% of the population are carriers of a genetic mutation that has a large effect on cancer risk and these cause less than 3–10% of cancer. Some of these syndromes include: certain inherited mutations in the genes BRCA1 and BRCA2 with a more than 75% risk of breast cancer and ovarian cancer, and hereditary nonpolyposis colorectal cancer (HNPCC or Lynch syndrome), which is present in about 3% of people with colorectal cancer, among others.

Statistically for cancers causing most mortality, the relative risk of developing colorectal cancer when a first-degree relative (parent, sibling or child) has been diagnosed with it is about 2. The corresponding relative risk is 1.5 for lung cancer, and 1.9 for prostate cancer. For breast cancer, the relative risk is 1.8 with a first-degree relative having developed it at 50 years of age or older, and 3.3 when the relative developed it when being younger than 50 years of age.

Taller people have an increased risk of cancer because they have more cells than shorter people. Since height is genetically determined to a large extent, taller people have a heritable increase of cancer risk.

Physical agents

Some substances cause cancer primarily through their physical, rather than chemical, effects. A prominent example of this is prolonged exposure to asbestos, naturally occurring mineral fibers that are a major cause of mesothelioma (cancer of the serous membrane) usually the serous membrane surrounding the lungs. Other substances in this category, including both naturally occurring and synthetic asbestos-like fibers, such as wollastonite, attapulgite, glass wool and rock wool, are believed to have similar effects. Non-fibrous particulate materials that cause cancer include powdered metallic cobalt and nickel and crystalline silica (quartz, cristobalite and tridymite). Usually, physical carcinogens must get inside the body (such as through inhalation) and require years of exposure to produce cancer.

Physical trauma resulting in cancer is relatively rare. Claims that breaking bones resulted in bone cancer, for example, have not been proven. Similarly, physical trauma is not accepted as a cause for cervical cancer, breast cancer or brain cancer. One accepted source is frequent, long-term application of hot objects to the body. It is possible that repeated burns on the same part of the body, such as those produced by kanger and kairo heaters (charcoal hand warmers), may produce skin cancer, especially if carcinogenic chemicals are also present. Frequent consumption of scalding hot tea may produce esophageal cancer. Generally, it is believed that cancer arises, or a pre-existing cancer is encouraged, during the process of healing, rather than directly by the trauma. However, repeated injuries to the same tissues might promote excessive cell proliferation, which could then increase the odds of a cancerous mutation.

Chronic inflammation has been hypothesized to directly cause mutation. Inflammation can contribute to proliferation, survival, angiogenesis and migration of cancer cells by influencing the tumor microenvironment. Oncogenes build up an inflammatory pro-tumorigenic microenvironment.

Hormones

Some hormones play a role in the development of cancer by promoting cell proliferation. Insulin-like growth factors and their binding proteins play a key role in cancer cell proliferation, differentiation and apoptosis, suggesting possible involvement in carcinogenesis.

Hormones are important agents in sex-related cancers, such as cancer of the breast, endometrium, prostate, ovary and testis and also of thyroid cancer and bone cancer. For example, the daughters of women who have breast cancer have significantly higher levels of estrogen and progesterone than the daughters of women without breast cancer. These higher hormone levels may explain their higher risk of breast cancer, even in the absence of a breast-cancer gene. Similarly, men of African ancestry have significantly higher levels of testosterone than men of European ancestry and have a correspondingly higher level of prostate cancer. Men of Asian ancestry, with the lowest levels of testosterone-activating androstanediol glucuronide, have the lowest levels of prostate cancer.

Other factors are relevant: obese people have higher levels of some hormones associated with cancer and a higher rate of those cancers. Women who take hormone replacement therapy have a higher risk of developing cancers associated with those hormones. On the other hand, people who exercise far more than average have lower levels of these hormones and lower risk of cancer. Osteosarcoma may be promoted by growth hormones. Some treatments and prevention approaches leverage this cause by artificially reducing hormone levels and thus discouraging hormone-sensitive cancers.

Autoimmune diseases

There is an association between celiac disease and an increased risk of all cancers. People with untreated celiac disease have a higher risk, but this risk decreases with time after diagnosis and strict treatment, probably due to the adoption of a gluten-free diet, which seems to have a protective role against development of malignancy in people with celiac disease. However, the delay in diagnosis and initiation of a gluten-free diet seems to increase the risk of malignancies. Rates of gastrointestinal cancers are increased in people with Crohn's disease and ulcerative colitis, due to chronic inflammation. Also, immunomodulators and biologic agents used to treat these diseases may promote developing extra-intestinal malignancies.

Pathophysiology

Genetics

Cancer is fundamentally a disease of tissue growth regulation. In order for a normal cell to transform into a cancer cell, the genes that regulate cell growth and differentiation must be altered.

The affected genes are divided into two broad categories. Oncogenes are genes that promote cell growth and reproduction. Tumor suppressor genes are genes that inhibit cell division and survival. Malignant transformation can occur through the formation of novel oncogenes, the inappropriate over-expression of normal oncogenes, or by the under-expression or disabling of tumor suppressor genes. Typically, changes in multiple genes are required to transform a normal cell into a cancer cell.

Genetic changes can occur at different levels and by different mechanisms. The gain or loss of an entire chromosome can occur through errors in mitosis. More common are mutations, which are changes in the nucleotide sequence of genomic DNA.

Large-scale mutations involve the deletion or gain of a portion of a chromosome. Genomic amplification occurs when a cell gains copies (often 20 or more) of a small chromosomal locus, usually containing one or more oncogenes and adjacent genetic material. Translocation occurs when two separate chromosomal regions become abnormally fused, often at a characteristic location. A well-known example of this is the Philadelphia chromosome, or translocation of chromosomes 9 and 22, which occurs in chronic myelogenous leukemia and results in production of the BCR-abl fusion protein, an oncogenic tyrosine kinase.

Small-scale mutations include point mutations, deletions, and insertions, which may occur in the promoter region of a gene and affect its expression, or may occur in the gene's coding sequence and alter the function or stability of its protein product. Disruption of a single gene may also result from integration of genomic material from a DNA virus or retrovirus, leading to the expression of viral oncogenes in the affected cell and its descendants.

Replication of the data contained within the DNA of living cells will probabilistically result in some errors (mutations). Complex error correction and prevention is built into the process and safeguards the cell against cancer. If a significant error occurs, the damaged cell can self-destruct through programmed cell death, termed apoptosis. If the error control processes fail, then the mutations will survive and be passed along to daughter cells.

Some environments make errors more likely to arise and propagate. Such environments can include the presence of disruptive substances called carcinogens, repeated physical injury, heat, ionising radiation or hypoxia.

The errors that cause cancer are self-amplifying and compounding, for example:

A mutation in the error-correcting machinery of a cell might cause that cell and its children to accumulate errors more rapidly.

A further mutation in an oncogene might cause the cell to reproduce more rapidly and more frequently than its normal counterparts.

A further mutation may cause loss of a tumor suppressor gene, disrupting the apoptosis signaling pathway and immortalizing the cell.

A further mutation in the signaling machinery of the cell might send error-causing signals to nearby cells.

The transformation of a normal cell into cancer is akin to a chain reaction caused by initial errors, which compound into more severe errors, each progressively allowing the cell to escape more controls that limit normal tissue growth. This rebellion-like scenario is an undesirable survival of the fittest, where the driving forces of evolution work against the body's design and enforcement of order. Once cancer has begun to develop, this ongoing process, termed clonal evolution, drives progression towards more invasive stages. Clonal evolution leads to intra-tumour heterogeneity (cancer cells with heterogeneous mutations) that complicates designing effective treatment strategies.

Characteristic abilities developed by cancers are divided into categories, specifically evasion of apoptosis, self-sufficiency in growth signals, insensitivity to anti-growth signals, sustained angiogenesis, limitless replicative potential, metastasis, reprogramming of energy metabolism and evasion of immune destruction.

Epigenetics

The classical view of cancer is a set of diseases that are driven by progressive genetic abnormalities that include mutations in tumor-suppressor genes and oncogenes and chromosomal abnormalities. Later epigenetic alterations' role was identified.

Epigenetic alterations are functionally relevant modifications to the genome that do not change the nucleotide sequence. Examples of such modifications are changes in DNA methylation (hypermethylation and hypomethylation), histone modification and changes in chromosomal architecture (caused by inappropriate expression of proteins such as HMGA2 or HMGA1). Each of these alterations regulates gene expression without altering the underlying DNA sequence. These changes may remain through cell divisions, last for multiple generations and can be considered to be epimutations (equivalent to mutations).

Epigenetic alterations occur frequently in cancers. As an example, one study listed protein coding genes that were frequently altered in their methylation in association with colon cancer. These included 147 hypermethylated and 27 hypomethylated genes. Of the hypermethylated genes, 10 were hypermethylated in 100% of colon cancers and many others were hypermethylated in more than 50% of colon cancers.

While epigenetic alterations are found in cancers, the epigenetic alterations in DNA repair genes, causing reduced expression of DNA repair proteins, may be of particular importance. Such alterations are thought to occur early in progression to cancer and to be a likely cause of the genetic instability characteristic of cancers.

Reduced expression of DNA repair genes disrupts DNA repair. This is shown in the figure at the 4th level from the top. (In the figure, red wording indicates the central role of DNA damage and defects in DNA repair in progression to cancer.) When DNA repair is deficient DNA damage remains in cells at a higher than usual level (5th level) and cause increased frequencies of mutation and/or epimutation (6th level). Mutation rates increase substantially in cells defective in DNA mismatch repair or in homologous recombinational repair (HRR). Chromosomal rearrangements and aneuploidy also increase in HRR defective cells.

Higher levels of DNA damage cause increased mutation (right side of figure) and increased epimutation. During repair of DNA double strand breaks, or repair of other DNA damage, incompletely cleared repair sites can cause epigenetic gene silencing.

Deficient expression of DNA repair proteins due to an inherited mutation can increase cancer risks. Individuals with an inherited impairment in any of 34 DNA repair genes (see article DNA repair-deficiency disorder) have increased cancer risk, with some defects ensuring a 100% lifetime chance of cancer (e.g. p53 mutations). Germ line DNA repair mutations are noted on the figure's left side. However, such germline mutations (which cause highly penetrant cancer syndromes) are the cause of only about 1 percent of cancers.

In sporadic cancers, deficiencies in DNA repair are occasionally caused by a mutation in a DNA repair gene but are much more frequently caused by epigenetic alterations that reduce or silence expression of DNA repair genes. This is indicated in the figure at the 3rd level. Many studies of heavy metal-induced carcinogenesis show that such heavy metals cause a reduction in expression of DNA repair enzymes, some through epigenetic mechanisms. DNA repair inhibition is proposed to be a predominant mechanism in heavy metal-induced carcinogenicity. In addition, frequent epigenetic alterations of the DNA sequences code for small RNAs called microRNAs (or miRNAs). miRNAs do not code for proteins, but can "target" protein-coding genes and reduce their expression.

Cancers usually arise from an assemblage of mutations and epimutations that confer a selective advantage leading to clonal expansion. Mutations, however, may not be as frequent in cancers as epigenetic alterations. An average cancer of the breast or colon can have about 60 to 70 protein-altering mutations, of which about three or four may be "driver" mutations and the remaining ones may be "passenger" mutations.

Metastasis

Metastasis is the spread of cancer to other locations in the body. The dispersed tumors are called metastatic tumors, while the original is called the primary tumor. Almost all cancers can metastasize. Most cancer deaths are due to cancer that has metastasized.

Metastasis is common in the late stages of cancer and it can occur via the blood or the lymphatic system or both. The typical steps in metastasis are local invasion, intravasation into the blood or lymph, circulation through the body, extravasation into the new tissue, proliferation and angiogenesis. Different types of cancers tend to metastasize to particular organs, but overall the most common places for metastases to occur are the lungs, liver, brain and the bones.

Metabolism

Normal cells typically generate only about 30% of energy from glycolysis,[106] whereas most cancers rely on glycolysis for energy production (Warburg effect). But a minority of cancer types rely on oxidative phosphorylation as the primary energy source, including lymphoma, leukemia, and endometrial cancer. Even in these cases, however, the use of glycolysis as an energy source rarely exceeds 60%. A few cancers use glutamine as the major energy source, partly because it provides nitrogen required for nucleotide

(DNA,RNA) synthesis. Cancer stem cells often use oxidative phosphorylation or glutamine as a primary energy source.

Several studies have indicated that the enzyme sirtuin 6 is selectively inactivated during oncogenesis in a variety of tumor types by inducing glycolysis. Another sirtuin, sirtuin 3 inhibits cancers that depend upon glycolysis, but promotes cancers that depend upon oxidative phosphorylation.

A low-carbohydrate diet (ketogenic diet) has been sometimes been recommended as a supportive therapy for cancer treatment.

Cancer Diets

Peach Smoothie

Serves 2

Ingredients

- 1 medium fresh peach, peeled, pitted, and chopped
- ½ c skim milk

- 14 oz non-fat vanilla yogurt
- 1 c ice cubes
- ground cinnamon, to taste

Directions

1. Place peach, milk, yogurt, and ice in a blender. Blend until smooth. Turn off machine and scrape down the sides of the blender with a rubber spatula. Blend again.

2. Pour the mixture into 2 glasses and sprinkle each with a little cinnamon. Serve at once. (You can garnish with strawberries if you want to be fancy.)

Tips / Comments:

A quick refreshing drink for breakfast or an afternoon snack.If fresh fruit is not in season you may substitute your favorite frozen fruit.Just select a product that does not have added sugar.

Nutrition Facts (per serving): Calories (101); Total Fat (0 g); Saturated Fat

(0 g); Cholesterol (3 mg); Carbohydrate (3 g); Fiber (1 g); Protein (5 g); Sodium (65 mg)

English Muffin

Breakfast Pizza

Serves 1

Ingredients

- 2 Tbs reduced fat cream cheese
- 1 tsp reduced fat sour cream
- ½ English muffin
- 1 small ripe peach, peeled and sliced
- ½ tsp light brown sugar
- ground cinnamon, to taste

Directions

1. Preheat broiler.

2. In a small bowl, combine cream cheese and sour cream.

3. Spread evenly over English muffin half.

4. Arrange peach slices on top. Sprinkle with cinnamon and brown sugar.

5. Broil until cheese browns around edges, about 2 minutes.

6. Cut in half or quarters and eat warm.

Tips / Comments:

Select a whole grain, high-fiber English muffin for the biggest “bang for the buck”.

Nutrition Facts (per serving): Calories (185); Total Fat (7 g); Saturated Fat (4.3 g); Cholesterol (25 mg); Carbohydrate (25 g); Fiber (3 g); Protein (6 g); Sodium (258 mg)

Multi-bran Muffins

Makes 16

Ingredients

- 1 ½ c oat bran 1 Tbs baking powder
- 1 c wheat bran 1 tsp baking soda
- ¼ c orange juice 1 c Splenda brown sugar blend
- 1 c low-fat milk 1 Tbs cinnamon
- ½ c canola oil 1 tsp orange peel
- 1 c egg substitute 1 c raisins or craisins
- 1 c flour 1 c walnuts, chopped
- ½ c whole wheat flour ½ c cinnamon chips, optional

Directions

1. Spray muffin cups with cooking spray or line with muffin papers. Preheat oven to 375°F.

2. Combine first 6 ingredients (oat bran through egg substitute) in large bowl; let sit 5 minutes.

3. Combine next 7 dry ingredients (through orange peel) in another bowl. Add to bran mixture and stir just until combined.

4. Stir in raisins/craisins, nuts and chips if using. Scoop into muffin cups and bake for 18 minutes.

5. Let cool in pan for 5 minutes, then remove muffins to rack and cool completely.

Tips / Comments:

Can freeze in plastic sandwich bags. When you want to serve them, remove muffins from bag and place on a plate. Microwave for 20 seconds to defrost, turn the plate, and microwave for another 15 seconds.

Nutrition Facts (per muffin): Calories (244); Total Fat (12 g); Saturated Fat (1 g); Cholesterol (0.5 mg); Carbohydrate (30 g); Fiber (4 g); Protein (6 g); Sodium (208 mg)

Breakfast Sandwich

Serves 1

Ingredients

- 1 whole grain English muffin, split and toasted

- (I use Food for Life sprouted muffins, in the frozen food section)
- 1 frozen, pre-cooked sausage patty, heated in a microwave
- according to package instructions
- mustard

Directions

1. Spread toasted muffin with a little mustard, sandwich with the sausage and enjoy.

Tips / Comments:

This is a very fast breakfast that doesn't spike my blood sugar. Having quick meal ideas handy makes life easier!

Nutrition Facts (per serving): Calories (290); Total Fat (12 g); Saturated Fat (2.5 g); Cholesterol (35 mg); Carbohydrate (30 g); Fiber (6 g); Protein (18 g); Sodium (520 mg)

Northwest Berry Puff

serves 6

Ingredients

- 2 large eggs
- 1 large egg white
- ½ c fat-free milk
- ½ c all-purpose flour
- 1 Tbs sugar
- pinch salt
- 2 c fresh berries of your choice
- 1 Tbs powdered sugar
- cooking spray

Directions

1. Heat the oven to 400°F. Spray a 10 inch glass pie pan or oven-safe skillet with cooking spray.

2. Beat the eggs and egg white in a medium bowl. Whisk in the milk.Slowly whisk in the flour, sugar, and salt. Pour into the prepared pan and bake 15 minutes. Reduce the heat to

350°F and bake for 10 minutes longer, or until the batter is puffed and browned.

3. Remove from the oven and slide onto serving plate. Cover with the fruit (if strawberries are used, slice into bite-sized pieces) and dust with powdered sugar. Cut into 6 wedges and serve.

Nutrition Facts (per serving): Calories (110); Total Fat (2 g); Saturated Fat (1g); Cholesterol (71 mg); Carbohydrate (18 g); Fiber (2 g); Protein (5 g); Sodium (89 mg)

Mushroom Omelet

Serves 2

Ingredients

- 6 oz fresh mushrooms, such as
- shitake, portobello, or
- button
- 2 scallions, white parts only,
- thinly sliced

- ¼ tsp minced thyme
- ¼ tsp minced basil
- 1 Tbs chopped fresh flat-leaf
- parsley
- freshly ground pepper
- 8 oz liquid egg substitute
- 2 sprigs fresh parsley, for garnish
- cooking spray

Directions

1. Spray a small non-stick skillet with cooking spray and heat over high heat for 1 minute.

2. Add mushrooms and scallions and cook over high heat until mushrooms are just cooked through.

3. Remove to small bowl and add herbs and seasonings.

4. Spray same skillet with cooking spray and add half of egg substitute. Cook over medium heat, lifting the sides of the eggs to allow the uncooked eggs to flow under.

5. Once the omelet is lightly browned, carefully flip the omelet to brown the other side.

6. Spoon half the mushroom mixture onto the omelet and fold in half. Transfer to a plate and keep warm in a warm oven, covered with foil.

7. Repeat, making a second omelet. Place a sprig of parsley on each omelet.

Tips / Comments:

Substitute any vegetable for or in addition to the mushrooms. One of our favorites is to sauté red and orange baby peppers. They add beautiful color and taste wonderful.

Nutrition Facts (per serving): Calories (83); Total Fat (tr g); Saturated

Fat (tr g); Cholesterol (0 mg); Carbohydrate (6 g); Fiber (1 g); Protein (14 g); Sodium (205 mg)

Sausage Strata

Ingredients

- ¾ c shredded low- fat 2 c 1% milk
- cheddar cheese 1 lb chicken or turkey sausage
- 8 slices, good quality 1 ½ c egg substitute
- white bread, crusts cooking spray
- removed and cut into cubes
- 1 ½ c roasted tomatillo salsa (recipe follows)

Directions

1. Remove and discard sausage casing. Crumble and brown in non-stick skillet, stirring and breaking up with a wooden spoon. Transfer with a slotted spoon to a paper-towel lined plate.

2. Whisk together milk and egg substitute in a large bowl.

3. Coat a 9"x9" baking dish with cooking spray. Set aside ¼ cup shredded cheese, wrapped, in the refrigerator.

4. Layer 1/3 of the bread cubes in the dish. Top with half the sausage and ¼ cup of the cheese.

5. Pour 1 cup of the milk mixture over the top.

6. Repeat the layers. Add the last of the bread on top, and pour over the last of the egg and milk mixture.

7. Cover with the tomatillo salsa. Cover with plastic wrap and refrigerate overnight.

8. In the morning, heat the oven to 350°F. Uncover the casserole, and sprinkle the top with reserved ¼ cup shredded cheese.

9. Bake until strata is golden brown and bubbling, and a knife inserted in the center comes out clean, about 50-60 minutes.

10. Let rest for 10 minutes before serving.

Tips / Comments:

A wonderful do-ahead brunch casserole without all the fat and carbs. The salsa adds a real wow factor.

Nutrition Facts (per serving): Calories (199); Total Fat (4 g); Saturated Fat (1.6 g); Cholesterol (24 mg); Carbohydrate (21 g); Fiber (1 g); Protein (20 g); Sodium (689 mg)

Roasted Tomatillo Salsa

Ingredients

- 8 fresh tomatillos, husks removed
- 1 jalapeno pepper, stem and seeds removed
- 1 lemon, grate zest and juice
- cooking spray

Directions

1. Preheat oven to 350°F.
2. Place tomatillos and jalapeno on small baking sheet. Spritz with cooking spray. Roast 20-25 minutes, or until tomatillos are soft and golden.
3. Transfer tomatillos and jalapeno to food processor and process until smooth.
4. Add lemon zest and juice. Pulse to mix.
5. Refrigerate until ready to use.

Nutrition Facts : Eaten on its own the salsa has 13 calories and 3 g carbohydrate per ¼ c serving.

Eggs Tudor

Ingredients

- 2 Tbs unsalted butter, divided 8 jumbo black olives chopped
- 2 Tbs flour 8 eggs
- 1 c half and half ¼ c 1% milk
- dash of salt 1 c turkey ham, slivered
- ¼ tsp white pepper, divided ¾ c grated Swiss cheese, divided
- 1/8 tsp nutmeg 2 cherry tomatoes, halved

Directions

1. Preheat broiler.

2. Melt 1 tablespoon butter, stir in flour and gradually stir in half and half. Add dash of salt, ½ the pepper and nutmeg, cook stirring until the sauce boils and thickens. Stir in ½ cup Swiss cheese and chopped olives. Stir over low heat until the cheese melts.

3. Beat eggs and milk together, add the remaining pepper to the eggs. Melt remaining tablespoon of butter and add the egg mixture. Cook over low heat until the eggs are set, stirring occasionally from the bottom of the pan.

4. Arrange turkey ham on bottom of 9"x13" baking dish. Top with 8 tablespoons of the sauce. Layer eggs on top and then spoon the remaining sauce over top and sprinkle with remaining cheese.

5. Place under broiler and broil until the top is slightly browned. Garnish each with the ½ cherry tomato.

Tips / Comments:

A family holiday favorite. This one is a splurge so make sure to balance carbs and calories for the rest of the day !

Nutrition Facts (per serving): Calories (368); Total Fat (26.6 g); Saturated Fat (12 g); Cholesterol (485 mg); Carbohydrate (10.5 g); Fiber (0.6 g); Protein (22.1 g); Sodium (585 mg)

Low Carb Chocolate Lasagna Sugar-free Dessert (no-bake)

Low Carb Chocolate Lasagna is a great sugar-free chocolate dessert made with a chocolate cookie base, cream cheese layer, chocolate pudding and whipped cream. This large dessert is great for gatherings.

Ingredients

CHOCOLATE PUDDING

- 1 recipe Low Carb Chocolate Pastry Cream

CHOCOLATE COOKIE CRUST

- 2 cups almond flour (180 g)
- 1 cup Shredded Coconut (90 g)
- 1/3 cup cocoa powder (25 g) (sifted)
- 1/4 cup low carb sugar (Sukrin :1, Swerve, Lakanto, Besti)
- 6 tablespoons salted butter

WHIPPED CREAM

- 2 cups heavy cream (16 oz)
- 2 tablespoons erythritol, powdered
- 1 teaspoon stevia glycerite
- 1 teaspoon vanilla extract
- LIGHTENED CREAM CHEESE
- 8 ounces cream cheese, softened
- 2 tablespoons almond milk
- 3 tablespoons sugar free powdered sugar (Sukrin, Swerve, Lakanto, Besti)
- 1/8 teaspoon stevia glycerite
- 1 1/2 cup whipped cream to be folded in

GARNISH

- 4 squares Ghirardelli Midnight Reverie (grated)

Instructions

1. Make the Chocolate Pudding: Prepare the Low Carb Chocolate Pastry Cream and let it cool before continuing. *This can be made several days before.

2. Make the Chocolate Cookie Crust: Grind the unsweetened coconut, 1/2 cup at a time, in a coffee/spice grinder until fine in texture. Put the ground coconut into a medium bowl and add the sweetener, cocoa, and almond flour. Whisk together to combine. Melt the butter or coconut oil and pour over the ingredients. Combine to form a moist crumbly mixture.
3. Dump the ingredients into a 13x9 inch glass pyrex baking dish and lay a sheet of waxed paper over the mixture. First with your hands, then with a flat bottomed glass, press the chocolate crust mixture firmly into the dish. Remove the waxed paper and continue with the recipe or *bake in a preheated (350) oven for about 10 minutes and then let cool completely. *This can be made the day before.

ASSEMBLING THE LOW CARB CHOCOLATE LASAGNA:

4. Make the Whipped Cream: Whip the cream with the vanilla and sweeteners until stiff.

5. Cream Cheese Layer: Soften the cream cheese in the microwave and then using a hand mixer, whip it with the sweeteners and almond milk until nice and light. Adding 1/2 cup of whipped cream at a time, fold 1 1/2 cups of whipped cream into the cream cheese. Spread evenly over the base and refrigerate.
6. Chocolate Pudding Layer: With a hand mixer, whip the cold pudding. Spread over the cream cheese layer.
7. Whipped Cream Topping: Carefully, spread the remaining whipped cream over the chocolate pudding layer and refrigerate several hours.
8. To finish the dessert, grate chocolate or sift cocoa powder over the top.

Notes

This is a VERY large dessert and easily serves 16-24 people.

NOTE: Baking the bottom layer produces a shortbread-cookie-like texture: not baking, produces a sandier and softer textured bottom layer

Superfine Flours for the Keto Baker

Flours taken from almonds and coconuts, ground to a superfine consistency, are Urvashi Pitre's favorites. She calls almond flour "the stalwart workhorse for keto baking" and notes that it is filling, which helps you avoid overindulgence. Hilda Solares agrees, calling it "the easiest of all low-carb flours to work with." Make sure you get almond flour and not an almond meal, which is coarser.

Coconut flour is a lot drier than the almond variety, which means you need to use more liquid and/or eggs when baking with it. As Solares notes, "For those who are allergic to tree nuts, coconut flour can be a great option." Not only can neither almond nor coconut flour is substituted on a cup-for-cup basis for wheat flour, but the two also cannot be substituted for one another.

Berry Good

Love fruit but hate the carb counts? Berries are your friends: Besides being packed with vitamins and health-promoting phytonutrients, many berries contain healthy amounts of fiber, which lowers their net carb numbers. For example:

Blackberries—contain 8 grams of fiber with 6 grams of net carbs per cup

Red Raspberries—provide 8 grams of fiber with 7 grams of net carbs in each cup

Strawberries—2 grams of fiber for a reasonable 5 grams net carbs in each 1/2 cup (sliced)

Chocolate-Cheesecake Brownies

"These brownies need to be well-cooled before you start to devour them, as they can be a little soft and fudgy when hot," says Urvashi Pitre. "Of course, if you want soft and fudgy, don't let me stop you!" And don't let the 21-gram total carb count per brownie stop you either since the net carbs are only 2 grams.

Keto cooking spray

For the brownie batter:

- 1/2 cup sugar-free chocolate chips
- 8 tbsp (1 stick) unsalted butter
- 3 large eggs
- 1 tsp vanilla extract
- 1/4 cup Swerve granulated sweetener

For the cheesecake batter:

- 8 oz full-fat cream cheese, cubed and softene
- 1 large egg
- 3 tbsp Truvía granulated sweetener
- 1 tsp vanilla extract

Instructions

1. Preheat the oven to 350°F. Grease an 8” square baking pan with cooking spray and line the bottom with parchment paper; set aside.
2. For the brownie batter: In a medium-sized, microwave-safe bowl, combine the chocolate chips and butter. Microwave on high for 1 minute, stopping and stirring once. Remove from the microwave and stir until all lumps have melted into the mixture (don’t continue to microwave).
3. In a large bowl, combine the eggs, vanilla, and sweetener. Beat with an electric mixer on medium-high until light and frothy. Slowly pour the melted chocolate mixture into the bowl, beating until well blended. Pour the batter into the prepared pan.
4. For the cheesecake batter: Combine all ingredients in a medium-sized bowl; beat with an electric mixer on medium-high until light and frothy. Pour the cheesecake batter on top of the brownie batter, and use a rubber scraper or butter knife to swirl the two batters together slightly.

5. Bake for 35 minutes, or until a knife inserted into the center comes out clean. (If you see the edges starting to cook faster than the rest of the brownie, cover the top loosely with foil.)
6. Cool in the pan on a wire rack for 10 minutes. Cut into 8 rectangles. Remove from the pan and cool completely on the rack.

Smoothie Recipes for Cancer Patients

Who doesn't like a smoothie? They are convenient and delicious. But for someone undergoing treatment for cancer, a smoothie is an especially great choice. When you're not feeling at your best and your appetite may be waning, a smoothie is a great way to take in some vital nutrients and stay hydrated – super important for maintaining your strength and feeling as well as possible while focusing on your treatment.

Why smoothies are good while undergoing cancer treatment

Loss of appetite is extremely common among those fighting cancer. Not only do some types of cancer cause appetite loss themselves, but common treatments also reduce appetite as part of their side effects.

Furthermore, some people may complain of sensitivity to certain smells or textures that turn them off of food. Smoothies can be a good way to partially overcome that challenge and still ensure proper nutrition.

That being said, it can be easy to get into a smoothie rut. We've scoured the internet to bring you a list of five smoothies to add to your rotation. B

Be sure to talk to your medical team about whether or not fresh fruits and veggies are a good option for you if you happen to have a low white blood cell count!

Banana Almond Butter Smoothie

This smoothie recipe from Real Simple Good combines four simple ingredients to create a delicious smoothie that is great as-is or that can easily be combined with your other favorite ingredients for a custom smoothie masterpiece. This recipe calls for bananas, which are a great source of fiber and potassium, as well as almond butter – a great source of protein and fat when you aren't feeling up to a steak dinner.

Rounded out with coconut milk (another good source of fat) and cinnamon, we'd be surprised if this smoothie doesn't quickly become one of your favorites.

Carrot Ginger Turmeric Smoothie

The anti-inflammatory properties of ginger and turmeric combined with carotenoid-rich carrots make Minimalist Baker's smoothie recipea slam dunk, particularly if you've been dealing with nausea. Most of the ingredients in this smoothie are also great for fortifying your immune system … And it looks so pretty!

High-Fiber Broccoli Smoothie for Kids

Okay, this smoothie proclaims to be specifically for kids. But don't rule it out if you happen to be an adult. If there's one thing I know to be true, it's that recipes targeted for kids typically taste 300% better than the stuff they try to get us adults to drink.

Loaded with broccoli, avocado and flax meal, this smoothie gets its delicious flavor and pretty color from cherries, banana and pomegranate juice.

Refreshing Watermelon Smoothie

This smoothie recipe from Live Eat Learn combines the hydrating qualities of watermelon and cucumber with fresh mint to create a delicious smoothie recipes for cancer patientssummertime smoothie. And given the hot weather in Phoenix, this may end up being one of your favorites to whip up year round. Furthermore, since mint is known to help settling stomachs and with other digestive issues, it may be a great option for cancer patients having issues with nausea or indigestion. But be aware, this smoothie is definitely light in the calories department.

Chocolate Peanut Butter Cup Smoothie

This smoothie recipe's impressive calorie requirements as a result of her cystic fibrosis. However, many cancer patients also struggle to meet their daily calorie quota. This recipe is a delicious, simple way to make headway while ensuring vital nutrients are making up caloric intake.

Furthermore, this recipe offers the flexibility of using whole cow's milk or substituting for coconut milk or a favorite nut milk for those with lactose sensitivities. Calling for chia seeds or flax seeds for added fiber, this recipe checks off a lot of boxes on many cancer patients' lists!

How Broccoli Fights Cancer

Studies show that there are compounds in cruciferous vegetables known as isothiocyanates that fight cancer.

However, as far as we know, these compounds are only present in raw or very gently cooked cruciferous vegetables. So, that's why this recipe uses gently blanched and frozen broccoli florets.

It's also easier to hide the flavor of frozen broccoli as opposed to fresh broccoli. And, the frozen florets even help to thicken the smoothie.

Recipe Steps

Step One

The first step of this recipe is to gather up your ingredients. The base of the smoothie is made from hemp seeds and water.

Step Two

Combine all of the ingredients in the base of a high-speed blender like a Blendtec or a Vitamix. Blend on high for just about 45 seconds, or until the smoothie is thick and creamy.

Step Three

Divide the smoothie between two glasses and serve immediately. You can store any leftovers in the refrigerator for up to 2 days.

Anti-Cancer Breakfast Smoothie

Description

This Anti-Cancer Green Breakfast Smoothie includes frozen broccoli florets, and other healthy ingredients. This recipe is vegan and dairy-free.

ingredients

- 1/4 cup hemp seeds
- 3 cups filtered water
- 1 ripe banana, frozen
- 1 cup frozen strawberries
- 1/4 cup frozen mango chunks

- 2 cups fresh salad greens or lightly steamed kale, spinach, or collard greens
- 5 fresh mint leaves
- 2 tablespoons cocoa powder
- 1 cup frozen raw broccoli florets
- juice of one lime

instructions

1. Combine hemp seeds and water in the base of a high-speed blender like a Vitamix or Blendtec.
2. Next, add the frozen banana, frozen strawberries, and frozen mango chunks, greens, mint, cocoa powder, broccoli, and lime juice.
3. Place the lid on the blender and blend until smooth, about 45 seconds.
4. Serve immediately.

notes

You can store any leftovers in a tightly-sealed container in the refrigerator for up to 2 days.

Category: Breakfast

Method: High-Speed Blender

Cuisine: American

Blueberry Blast Smoothie

Smoothies have many benefits beyond good taste; they can help you eat more fruits and vegetables, the foundation of a cancer-protective diet. Frozen blueberries are the secret to the milkshake-like consistency of this smoothie. Rich in fiber, anthocyanins and ellagic acid, these little fruits are being studied for their ability to inhibit the formation of carcinogens.

Ingredients

- 2 cups frozen unsweetened blueberries (do not thaw)
- 1/2 cup orange juice (calcium-fortified preferred)
- 3/4 cup low-fat or nonfat vanilla yogurt
- 1/2 medium frozen banana
- 1/2 tsp. pure vanila extract
- Makes 2 servings. Per serving: 220 calories, 2.5 g total fat (1 g saturated fat, 0 g trans fat), 5 mg cholesterol, 46 g carbohydrates, 6 g protein, 5 g dietary fiber, 65 mg sodium, 35 g sugar.

Directions

1. Place blueberries, orange juice, yogurt, banana and vanilla into blender.
2. Cover securely and blend for 30 to 35 seconds or until thick and smooth. For thinner smoothies, add more juice; for thicker smoothies, add more frozen fruit.
3. Pour into 2 glasses and serve immediately.

Notes

Don’t have frozen blueberries? Try frozen pineapple, cherries or mango.

www.ingramcontent.com/pod-product-compliance
Ingram Content Group UK Ltd.
Pitfield, Milton Keynes, MK11 3LW, UK
UKHW021655190726
13853UKWH00001B/265

9 798533 181624